THE GRAND UNIFIED THEORY OF PHYSIOLOGY

Dr. OMKAR PRASAD BAIDYA

PRACHI PUBLISHING

ISBN : 9788199146631
Edition : First, September 2025
Title : The Grand Unified Theory of Physiology
Author : Dr. Omkar Prasad Baidya

Published by

PRACHI PUBLISHING

An Imprint of **Taneesha and Prachi NextGen Publication**

Registered Office: Sunil Complex, 2nd Floor, Vijay Nagar,
Western Kutchery Road, Meerut - 250002, Uttar Pradesh, India
Website : www.prachipublishing.com
E-mail : help@prachipublishing.com
Phone : 0121 453 0364

Printed by :
Manipal Technologies Limited, Bengaluru - 560001, Karnataka

Dedication

Dedicated to Lord Brahma, Lord Shiva, Lord Vishnu, my Gurudev Sri Sri Swami Swarupananda Paramahamsa Dev, my respected father Sri Subhash Chandra Baidya and late mother Srimati Sabita Baidya

Preface

This book is a scientific book based on the physiological systems of human body. Here, in this book, I have tried to integrate all the systemic functions under the platform of mathematical physiology and physiological principles.

I tried to show that all systems of human physiology, are interlinked so as to design an equation which unifies parameters of all the systems of the human body. In this book, I tried my best to develop an integrated theory of physiology, where all systemic parameters are integrated to design an equation which can explain all the systemic functions of the human body. Here, in this book some preexisting scientific formulae and physiological principles of all physiological systems are analyzed in depth and has been correlated with the parameters of other systems of the human body. Besides, new functions and empirical formulas has been created wherever found to be needed based on preexisting physiological literature and scientific facts. Besides, some hypothesis has been made and new equations has been created which can estimate the parameters of all other systems of the human body. Finally, an equation has been designed which can unify all the systems of the human physiology including unification of electromagnetism, gravity and quantum mechanics and final modelled equation can be defined as the grand unified theory of physiology.

I would like to acknowledge my father who is continuous source of inspiration behind writing this book. I am grateful to the publisher who have guided me in publishing this book.

14th September 2025.
Kolkata
Dr. Omkar Prasad Baidya

Contents

Introduction

Physiology is the subject which deals with the study of normal function of living organisms including human body. Since, human beings are the natures best creation due to his highly developed brain and other systems of the body, human physiology systems become very complex as they develop with time under the process of organic evolution and nature-human body interaction guided by body demand and necessities depending on the adverse situation or external environment variation. Human physiological system consists of cardiovascular system, central nervous system, excretory system, respiratory system, endocrine system, reproductive system, neuromuscular system, gastrointestinal system, immune system, hematological system, etc. Each system consists of organs which are again composed of tissues and cellular architecture or cells. The common mission of the systems, or the organs and the cells is to work in such a manner that it creates a physiological environment inside human body necessary for survival, existence and maintenance of life and species in this planet earth. If we look deeper, if we want to make the human body active, it needs the electrical activities to happen in human body, and for that it needs the generation of bioelectricity in each cell and this give all cells their electrical properties which are nothing but due to positive and negative ions and their movements inside and outside of the cell membrane via pumps or channels which may or may not require ATP for their working. These electrical properties of specialized cardiac cells give its contractile nature and conductivity, excitability etc and all these together make the heart electrically active and pumping organ, which pumps blood to whole human body and help in survival of all the tissues and organs, cells of the human body by supplying nutrition, oxygen, etc and removal of toxic metabolites like CO2, lactic acid etc. Thus, it can be seen that biophysical phenomenon of bioelectricity development in cardiac cells is responsible for making the heart work in favor of human circulation by generation of force of contraction of heart. Cardiac muscle has both electrical and mechanical properties which help them in doing their function. The force of contraction generation of heart is based on the starling law of heart i.e the force of contraction of heart is directly proportional to initial length of cardiac muscle fiber. It is the heart which supply blood to all organs of the body and maintains the circulation to all organs and cardiac function is responsible for maintenance of CVS parameters like HR, BP, CO etc. Similarly, respiratory system plays important role in gaseous exchange and also for the oxygenation of blood and the various parameters of respiratory system consists of PACO2, VT etc. Similarly, all systems of human body have their individual functions so as to help human beings in their survival. Till now no such theory exist which unifies all physiological systemic parameters under the platform of mathematics and physiological law and principles. In this book, I will try to integrate all the functions of the physiological systems of the human body and design an equation which can integrate all the functional parameters of the systems of the human physiology.

What is the Grand unified theory of physiology?

In physics, there is a grand unified theory or theory of everything which unifies all four fundamental forces of nature like gravity, electromagnetism, strong nuclear force and weak nuclear force in a single set of equations and it is also known as theory of everything in physics. In physiology, there is no such theory at present. But, by grand unified theory of physiology, I mean to refer to the unified theory of physiology and this theory is formed by integrating the important parameters of all the physiological systems of the human body in a single set of equations, that directly or indirectly can explain the physiological changes in the human body based on the various changes in the physiological parameters and can show the interdependence and interlinking of the all the systems of the human physiology. Infact, all the systems of physiology, work interdependent manner in favor of maintaining the physiological state of the body. Nature has interlinked all the systems so that they together can play role in homeostasis of the body, help in physiological stability of the human body, create an internal environment suitable for survival of all the tissues and cells of the body, and thus helps in the maintenance of life and survival of the human body. Every system has some important parameters which play important role in the reflecting the efficacy and stability of the system. For example, in case of CVS, blood pressure, cardiac output, heart rate etc reflect whether the system is working effectively or not. Similarly, GFR shows the efficacy of excretory system. In this unified theory, I have tried to integrate all the systems of physiology by mathematically correlating all the important parameters of each system and thus if all the important parameters of all the physiological systems of human biological system can be correlated in a single equation that unified theory of physiology can be proved. In physics, grand unified theory refers to the integration or unification of all the fundamental forces of nature and in physiology, it refers to the unifications of all the complex systems of the human physiological system. In physiology, there are very less or limited universal laws and principles that govern the physiological phenomenon. This is because, physiological systems are closed systems and biological systems and they work in optimum pH, temperature, certain oxygen level, pco2 level, enzyme level, hormone level, certain electrolytes concentrations etc. Beyond these optimum values, either heart muscle will start failing, or proteins start degeneration, internal environment becomes unsuitable for survival of tissues, cells, organs and survival and life is affected. Thus, laws of physics and physical world even if applicable in physical world, may not be full-fledged applicable in physiological system which is mostly a biological system with many limitations. Hence, there are few laws and principle that govern the physiological system compared to physics and chemistry. However, scientist apply some laws of physics, biochemistry to explain many biophysical phenomena which also have limitations in biological systems. In this grand unified theory of physiology, I have tried to integrate or unify all the important parameters of each systems which reflects their functions using mathematical equations of biophysics, physiological principles etc. in a single equation. At present, there is not any single grand unified theory of physiology that exist in literature to the best of my knowledge. Hence, this theory will be first of its kind in the world and this is my effort to integrate all the systems in a single equation. In one of my books "Natures design of human physiological system", I have shown that how haemopoietic system interlinks with all other systems to maintain physiological stability of the human body. Thus, in this theory, I tried to integrate all the physiological systems and their parameters under the platform of mathematics and physics and derive an equation which includes all the parameters of the physiological systems of the human body. Lastly, I have also tried to unify two fundamental forces i.e gravity and electromagnetism along with quantum mechanics under the common platform of physiology so as to make this theory a grand unified theory of physiology. As per the physiology literature till now, there is not a single equation which can integrate all the systemic functions and hence, I have tried my best to design a mathematical model so as to unifies all the systemic functions in a single equation.

Nature and Unification of all the physiological systems

Nature is the greatest scientist as it has created all living creatures out of the basic biologic components and entities of life gradually under the process of organic evolution. Besides, nature has created human beings as the biologically superior and developed species on the earth and all these are not only due to developed brain and central nervous system but also due to complex and developed physiological systems of the human body and all these ultimately makes him adjustable to various adverse situations like exercise, hypoxia, emergency, pregnancy, hunger, poverty, lack of food and water, diseases and illness. Due to highly developed brain and presence of prefrontal cortex, human beings are intelligent species on earth, they can have rational thinking, logical and mathematical capability, morality development, creative and visionary thinking, spirituality development, future predictive capacity and scientific aptitude and technological innovation. All the complex arrangements of the physiological system is to maintain the human survival, existence, species maintenance, and in favor of maintenance of life in this planet earth or beyond. In my book "Natures design of human physiological system", I have shown that how nature has designed complex physiological system so as to promote human survival, existence, stability of physiological system, and maintenance of life and species in the earth or beyond. I have also shown that nature is moral, rational, logical and do all the complex arrangement in favor of life maintenance, human survival, maintenance of physiological environment, inside and in favor of the benefit of the human species and also for the stability of the physiological state of human body. Nature has designed all physiological systems, structural organs, organ functions, physiological laws, principles, molecular pathway, biophysical molecules and their signaling pathway such that it leads to stability of human physiological system, benefits human biological systems, and also for the greater benefit of human body, survival, existence, and maintenance of internal homeostasis and also help human beings to survive in various adverse situations like pregnancy, hunger and water scarcity, starvation, hypoxia, deep sea diving, high altitude travel and adjustments, exercise, and in emergency situation like i.e fight, flight and fight. Also, I want to state that our nature has a moral intension, rational framework, and moral consciousness, and logical framework guided by which it designs all the complex system which are present uniformly in all the physiological system, maintenance of bioelectricity and maintenance and survival of human life directly and indirectly. One of the important natures design of human physiological system is that human body is functional under the phenomenon of interlinking of all the physiological systems of the human body. That means all the systems together help in the maintenance of physiological stability, maintenance of internal homeostasis and origin and maintenance of body's electrical activity or bioelectricity of life which ultimately help in the human survival, existence, maintenance of life and species in this earth or beyond.

Cardiovascular system and its interlinking with other physiological system

Cardiovascular system consists of heart and blood vessels. Heart generates force of contraction which generates the pumping activities and pump the blood in forward direction to all blood vessels and finally to whole body tissues and cells and allow them to survive and this pumping activity is due to electrical activities generates due to automaticity, excitability and conductivity of cardiac muscle both working myocardial cell and pace making tissues.

Cardiovascular system (CVS) and Central nervous system (CNS) interlinking:

1. CVS and CNS are interlinked and influence each other due to the nature design of human biological system. CVS supply O2, blood circulation, nutrition to brain cells and neuronal tissues of the CNS and remove toxins, Co2, metabolites, from the neuronal tissue and thus help in survival of the neuronal tissues, which cannot tolerate hypoglycemia and hypoxia for long time.

2. Brain consists of cardiac centers i.e VMC and CIC, which can control heart rate, cardiac output, Blood pressure by sympathetic and parasympathetic nervous system.

3. Baroreceptors present in the arch of aorta part of CVS is connected to Higher centers like NTS i.e nucleus tractus solitarius via 9th and 10th cranial nervous and this connection controls the baroreceptors reflex and help in short term regulation of blood pressure.

4. Baroreceptor reflex connects heart and blood vessels to brainstem and plays important role in BP regulation.

5. Sympathetic and parasympathetic nervous supply to blood vessels help in vasoconstriction and vasodilatation of the blood vessels depending upon the vascular beds and thus controls the vascular resistance and blood pressure of the systemic arteries and also maintain vascular smooth muscle tone.

6. Sympathetic and parasympathetic also supply the venous system, controls the vasomotor tone and help in the maintenance of venous return to heart.

7. Astrocytes of CNS and endothelial lining of the blood vessels supplying the brain together maintains the integrity of the blood-brain-barrier which prevent unnecessary entry of toxic substances and molecules from entering into CNS.

8. CVS along with blood vessels form the brain vasculature which supply blood to brain and maintain perfusion pressure and blood pressure, which forms the basis of tissue perfusion brain.

9. In clinical practice, many vascular diseases like ischemia, thrombosis, hemorrhage, etc leads to neuronal damage due to neuronal hypoxia and this condition may be defined as stroke or cerebrovascular accident.

10. Simliarly, brainstem stroke or trauma to the brainstem which contain cardiovascular centers, can affect the cardiac activity.

11. Similarly, cardiogenic shock, heart failure, etc effect the normal functioning of brain, cognitive function and the overall brain health.

CVS and blood interlinking

1. CVS i.e heart pumps blood through blood vessels, which supply oxygen, nutrition, etc to all tissues of the body.

2. Heart pumps blood and helps in the generation of blood flow or velocity of blood which is responsible for tissue perfusion and due to free flow of blood and smoothness of inner lining of blood vessels, blood clotting dies not occur physiologically.

3. Atrium secretes ANP, BNP i.e atrial natriuretic peptide which act as natriuretic peptide and promote $Na+$ excretion via kidney along with water and maintain blood volume and sodium concentration.

4. Blood supply nutrition, O2 to heart muscle and cardiac tissue and remove CO2, lactic acid from cardiac tissue and helps in survival of cardiac tissue.

5. Blood maintains sufficient concentration of sodium, k+, Calcium, magnesium etc in the ECF which help in the cardiac contraction maintenance.

6. Cardiac or heart generates force of contraction which helps in maintaining cardiac output, blood pressure, along with the blood volume present in the ECF fluid.

7. In vascular injury, platelet of the blood helps in the thrombus formation in the injured area by formation of platelet plug and there after clot formation due to clotting factors activation which occurs due to clotting factors in the blood and thus bleeding is stopped.

8. Plasma proteins and RBC present in the blood are responsible for the blood viscosity which is associated with the increase in peripheral resistance of the blood vessels and when peripheral resistance is increased, blood pressure will be increased.

9. Potassium and calcium ions and other ionic level in the blood is responsible for cardiac excitability, contractility etc.

10. Together, CVS and blood play's important role in internal homeostasis mechanism for Ph, temp, and fluid balance.

11. Heart pumps the blood along with the immune system like WBC, ILs, T4 cells, antibodies, complement systems, etc and thus help in the immune defense mechanism of the body.

CVS and respiratory system interlinking

1. Heart and lung are interconnected via pulmonary circulation. Heart pumps due to which deoxygenated blood is transported from right ventricle to pulmonary circulation via pulmonary arteries and finally to pulmonary capillaries, which forms the respiratory membrane barrier along with the other layer of respiratory membrane barrier along with the other layer of respiratory membrane and promotes gaseous exchange in the pulmonary alveolar pulmonary gas exchange zone and this helps in the oxygenation of the deoxygenated blood from the right side of the heart and right ventricle.

2. After the oxygenation and gaseous exchange in alveolo-capillaries barrier the oxygenated blood is carried back to left atrium via 4 pulmonary veins, which are also component of vascular system of the CVS and thus pulmonary circulation i.e pulmonary arteries, veins connect heart and lung.

3. CVS plays important role supplying oxygen, nutrition, to lung parenchyma and remove the toxic metabolites from the lung tissues and thus help in the survival of the lung tissues.

4. Whenever there is an increase or decrease of BP, it will be sensed by baroreceptor reflex and thus with the help of vasomotor center and other Cardiovascular center, it helps in bringing back the BP to normal level and at the same time respiratory centers are also stimulated or inhibited as observed by the change of the respiratory rate and the depth of respiration. Thus, it can be cardiovascular centers are interlined with respiratory centers and hence if any of the two is stimulated, another center will also be involved.

5. Ventilation/perfusion ratio is associated with perfusion which is nothing but the cardiac output and this reaction is very important in controlling the gaseous exchange at lung.

CVS and excretory system interlinking

1) CVS is associated with development of PGc or capillary hydrostatic pressure of the Starling force (net), which depends upon Systemic arterial pressure and all these finally contribute to the GFR formation via kidney.

2) Kidney help in the regulation of long-term control of Blood pressure via RAS system.

3) Kidney plays important role in regulation of blood pressure via renin angiotensin system.

4) Atrium secretes ANP which acts on the kidney to excrete Na+, H20 through kidney and helps in balance in ECF.

5) Kidney plays important role in electrolyte homeostasis and water balance in the ECF.

6) CVS, kidney and blood together help in the maintenance of electrolyte balance in the ECF.

7) CVS along with renal blood vessels supply blood to kidneys and other organs and structure of excretory system and also remove the toxic metabolites via renal vein and venous system of the excretory system and thus help in the survival of the excretory system organs directly or indirectly.

8) Kidney maintenance electrolytes concentration, [Na], [K], pH and other positive ions and negative ions in blood, which creates sufficient necessary atmosphere for contraction of cardiac tissue or heart to generate force of contraction and other cardiac function.

9) High Blood pressure, stimulates baroreceptors reflex which decrease VMC, increase Cardiac inhibitory centre, and lower HR, CO, BP and also effect respiratory centre and thus effect rate and depth of

respiration.

10) Several antihypertensives drugs like furosemide, or loop diuretics acts on kidneys to excrete Na+, K+, Cl ions, and water to lower Blood pressure directly or indirectly.

11) Diseases of heart and blood vessels like high BP can affect and harm kidneys and GFR directly and indirectly.

12) Low BP or shock like cardiogenic shock also effects kidneys blood flow or renal blood flow and perfusion pressure and this effect urine output and even leads to acute kidney failure (AKF) due to less blood supply to kidneys.

CVS and GIT interlinking

1) CVS supply blood to GIT organs and promotes their survival and help in the performing their normal function.

2) GIT help in absorption of nutrients like amino acid, glucose, [Na], [K], positive ions, negative ions, fatty acids, along H20, and thus help in maintenance of blood volume, and blood pressure and cardiac output.

3) GIT also absorbs [Na], [K], positive ions, negative ions, fatty acids, along with H20 and thus helps in maintenance of extracellular electrolyte balance, and thus electrolytes help in the cardiac electrical activities.

4) Liver produces albumin and plasma proteins which help in the maintenance of blood viscosity and this blood viscosity, maintains peripheral resistance and Blood pressure.

CVS and reproductive system interlinking

1. CVS supply blood to reproductive organs and help in the survival and maintenance of health, the reproductive organs, and their normal functions.

2. Hormones like NA, Adrenaline, Epinephrine, norepinephrine, that effect heart also effects the reproductive activity.

3. Reproductive hormones like oestrogen have vasodilation effect on the cardiovascular system and maintains CVS health and prevents risk of MI, cardiac disease in women and female.

4. Testosterone also has huge impact on CVS by increase BP, increase in lipid profile.

5. During menstruation, there occurs menstrual cycle that influence, CVS function like change in blood pressure.

6. During pregnancy, some complications like pregnancy induced hypertension occurs, which effect cardiovascular health and maternal health etc.

CVS and endocrine system linking

1) Many neuroendocrine secretions like noradrenaline, adrenaline etc has immense effect on the inotropic state of heart and also on the other effects on the cardiac function like excitability, conductivity, chronotropic effect and all these neurotransmitters and neurosecretions effect HR, BP, CO etc.

2) Many hormones like thyroid hormones have inotropic effect on the heart and this action is also known to be permissive to adrenaline and noradrenaline.

3) Hormones like ADH help in the H20 absorption via kidney tubules and rhus help in the maintenance of water volume of ECF and bloods volume, which ultimate effect BP.

4) Hormones like cortisol, mineralocorticoids, aldosterone, produced from adrenal gland, helps in the sodium and water from the kidney and thus help in the maintenance of sodium, H20, content of ECF volume which directly and indirectly maintains blood volume, plasma osmolarity and blood pressure.

5) Atrium secretes a hormone called ANP which helps in Na+, H20, excretion via kidney and thus helps in the maintaining of Na+, H20 level in the blood and hence balances Na+, H20 volume of ECF and also maintains BP and Cardiac output.

6) Kidney secretes an hormone known as erythropoietin which

produce RBC production and this RBC helps in the viscosity of blood, which effect the peripheral vascular resistance and which final impact blood pressure, which is an important parameter of the cardiovascular system.

7) Renin produced by kidney, can play important role in blood pressure regulation via renin angiotensin system.

8) Oestrogen hormone has a vasodilatory effect on the blood vessels, and it also protects female from cardiovascular risk factors and prevent many cardiovascular diseases like myocardial infarction.

9) Cortical produced from adrenal cortex, increases vascular responsive to catecholamines and contributes to hypertension.

10) Diseases like pheochromocytoma occurs due to excess catecholamines which are also called neuroendocrine secretions and this tumour of adrenal medulla, leads to hypertension, tachycardia.

11) In hyperthyroidism, there is excess production and secretion of thyroid hormones from the thyroid gland and in this disease, there occurs tachycardia and arrythmia.

12) Similarly, in case of hypothyroidism, there occurs decrease in thyroid hormones, which ultimately leads to bradycardia, hypotension and pericardial effusion etc.

13) In Cushing syndrome, there is excessive secretion of cortisol, which ultimately leads to hypertension, atherosclerosis and thus leads to diseases of cardiovascular system.

14) In diabetes malleus, which occurs due to lack of insulin production or insulin resistance, there occurs metabolic dysregulation which effect hyperlipemia, atherosclerosis and hypertension and all these increases the risk of silent myocardial infarction and stroke, both of which are vascular disease.

15) In conns syndrome, there occurs excess production of aldosterone which leads to hypertension, hypernatremia and hypokalaemia and these further leads to cardiovascular complications.

CVS and immune system interlinking

CVS and immune system are tightly interconnected. Their interaction and interconnection are essential for maintaining homeostasis responding to injury or infection and contribution to acute and chronic disease status like atherosclerosis and myocarditis.

1. CVS supply blood containing immune system i,e immune cells, complement system, antibodies to whole body organs, tissues and fight against foreign toxic invading agents in various parts of the body.
2. The immune system consists of inflammation which is a central feature of many cardiovascular diseases. Inflammation leads to atherosclerosis, myocarditis and vasculitis.
3. Cytokine release affects vascular tone, myocardial function and can cause systemic effects eg sepsis.
4. Auto Immune diseases can target cardiac tissues and leads to rheumatic heart diseases, lupus myocarditis.
5. Atherosclerosis occurs due to low grade inflammation and this atherosclerosis that occurs leads to vascular diseases like MI, stroke.
6. Besides, all immune cells can affect cardiovascular system and even leads to cardiovascular diseases.
7. Macrophage proliferation can lead to atherosclerosis plaque formation and rupture.
8. T lymphocyte secret pro-inflammatory cytokine, involved in myocarditis.
9. B lymphocytes, produce antibodies can participate in autoimmunity.
10. Neutrophils involved in acute inflammation and vascular injury.
11. Mast cells release histamine which effect vascular permeability.
12. Dendritic cells act as antigen presenting cells in atherosclerosis.
13. Autoimmune diseases like SLE can affect cardiovascular diseases and can leads to pericarditis, myocarditis, atherosclerosis etc.
14. Rheumatoid arthritis, an autoimmune disease increases the risk of MI, stroke.

15. Vasculitis like Kawasaki, Takayasu arteritis leads to vessel inflammation like stenosis, aneurysm.

16. Covid19 is a viral infection that can leads to systemic inflammation that myocarditis, thrombosis, endothelial damage.

17. Endothelial cells can act as an interface between CVS and immune system and thus any systemic inflammation can lead to vascular dysfunction and thus leads to thrombosis.

18. In immune system disorder and inflammation, heart may be targeted for eg in myocarditis, there is autoimmune attack on heart.

19. In pericarditis, there is immune attack on pericardium as seen in SLE.

20. The immune system regulates and responds to cardiovascular changes especially through inflammation.

21. Inflammation contributes to plaque development, endothelial dysfunction and vascular injury.

22. Autoimmune disease can affect heart and blood vessel.

23. Many drugs that treat cardiovascular diseases acts by modulating immune systems like anti-TNF, IL-1 blocker etc.

Interlinking with CNS with other systems of human physiology

CNS consists of brain and spinal cord and peripheral nerves and all together comes nervous system. Brain has many lobes and parts like cerebral corte, midbrain, limbic system, cerebellum, brainstem (midbrain, pons, medulla oblangata). Prefrontal cortex (PFC) is the most developed part of human brain due to which human beings becomes most intelligent due to which human beings becomes most intelligent and developed species in the earth. Due to PFC, human beings can do mathematical calculation, logical thinking, visionary thinking, predictive capacity, societal, social rational, rational behaviour, moral decision making etc and thus due to highly developed brain human beings can have emotional intelligence, spiritual intelligence and thus human beings can be spirituality and scientifically advanced species in the world. Let's see nervous system has interlinking with other systems of the body.

CNS and CVS interlinking

Now, nature has interlinked CNS and cardiovascular system and practically also they are deeply interlinked, working together to regulate blood pressure, heart rate, vascular tone and to respond to stress, exercise or injury.

1. Autonomic nervous system, a division of CNS is the primary controller of cardiovascular system.

2. Sympathetic nervous activity has immense effect on the heart by increasing the heart rate, cardiac output, blood pressure, conductivity, inotropic property and leads to

vasoconstriction in most of the vascular bed.

3. Parasympathetic nervous system lowers heart rate, cardiac output, BP by its negative inotropic effect, negative chronotropic effect, dromotropic effect and negative bathmotropic effect.

4. Brains cardiovascular centres such as Nucleus tractus solitarius, cardiac stimulatory area, cardiac inhibitory are etc. hypothalamus etc can play important role in blood pressure and heart rate regulation via the baroreceptor reflex input and sympathetic, parasympathetic output.

5. Various reflex arcs work by interlinking of CNS and CVS as for example baroreceptor reflex, chemoreceptor reflex, etc. Baroreceptors is present in great arteries; sense blood pressure change and transmit via 9th and 10th Cranial nerves to cardiovascular centres and thus help in controlling the blood pressure, respiration, and heart rate.

6. CNS regulates heart and blood vessels during stress.

7. Various diseases like stroke, CVA, ischemic stroke, haemorrhagic stroke etc occurs due to vascular pathology like endothelial injury, and other factors like hypertension and hyperlipidaemia.

CNS and Endocrine system interlinking

CNS and endocrine system are closely interlinked forming the system called neuroendocrine system. This neuro endocrine system helps in growth, metabolism, response to stress, reproduction, homeostasis, through neural control of hormone release and hormonal feedback to the brain.

1. Hypothalamus is a neuroendocrine master of human brain and connects brain to endocrine system. It releases hormones like TRH, CRH, GnRH, dopamine etc and regulates pituitary gland.
2. Hypothalamus directly releases hormones like ADH, oxytocin via posterior pituitary neuronal endings into blood and regulates various activities in the human system.
3. Hypothalamus controls other glandular secretions via hypothalamic -pituitary axis.
4. Hormones secreted from hypothalamus also acts on various organs of the body.
5. Brain contains a structure called hypothalamus which secretes many hormones and control pituitary and other endocrine glans of the human body.
6. ADH secreted from hypothalamus and posterior pituitary plays important role in water regulation of the body.
7. Catecholamines like adrenaline, noradrenaline etc produce from sympathetic nerve endings of adrenal medulla and these catecholamines are also called neuroendocrine secretions which have huge impact on the heart, blood vessels by effecting BP, CO and heart rate.
8. Thyroid hormones have immense effect on the central nervous system by maintaining neuronal growth and mental health.
9. Melatonin from pineal gland helps in the sleep wake cycle.
10. Insulin, T3, cortisol etc plays role in cognitive function.

CNS and reproductive system interlinking

1. Sympathetic and parasympathetic activity effect reproductive

activity directly and indirectly.

2. Many reproductive hormones like oestrogen, testosterone have impact on human mind, mood, cognition, function, social behaviour, and human nature.

3. CNS can influence hypothalamus which secretes GnRh and this hormone acts on pituitary to secrete LSH, FSH etc which acts a gonad (reproductive organs) to produce

testosterone and oestrogen etc which play important role in reproduction of human being.

4. CNS also plays important role in reproductive activity.

CNS and GIT system interlinking

1. Autonomic nervous system has immense impact on GIT motility and secretion. Sympathetic stimulation and activity lowers GI secretion and gi motility.

2. Parasympathetic activity and stimulation increase GI secretions and gi motility.

3. Hypothalamus have two important centres i.e feeding centres (ventromedial nucleus) and satiety centre (lateral hypothalamus). These two centres together play important role in food intake or feeding behaviour, which is an important mechanism of gastrointestinal system.

4. CNS via autonomic nervous system controls GI hormones secretion like gastrin and cholecystokinin which control digestion and absorption.

5. Gut brain axis can influence appetite, satiety and food preference and also food intake.

6. Any dysregulation of gut brain axis contributes to various GIT disorders like irritable bowel syndrome, IBD, GERD etc.

7. Gut microbiota influences production of NTs, hormones etc that impact CNS function.

CNS and excretory system interlinking

1. Brain and spinal cord controls micturition reflex i.e micturition reflex.
2. Pons and cerebral cortex have pontine micturition centre which coordinates urination.
3. Frontal lobe inhibits or can help in voluntary stoppage of urination.
4. Parasympathetic neurons stimulate detrusor muscle contraction.
5. Hypothalamus help in the secretion of ADH which help in the water absorption in kidney.
6. Hypothalamus controls thirst regulation which help in water intake.
7. CNS receives pain signals from the excretory system from excretory system.
8. Toxic accumulation of toxins like urea can effect brain as for example uremic encephalopathy.
9. Medulla and hypothalamus regulate excretion based on blood composition.
10. Hypothalamus also helps in internal homeostasis of the body.
11. Brain also plays role in BP regulation which can easily affect GFR.

CNS and respiratory system interlinking

1. Brainstem contains respiratory centres and bulb pontine respiratory group of neurons which controls the rate and depth of respiration
2. Respiratory centres in brain control respiration.
3. Chemoreceptors are connected to respiratory centres and can play important role in respiration.
4. Cerebral cortex plays important role in voluntary control of respiration if needed.
5. Limbic system plays important role in emotional control of

respiration.

6. Stroke may affect the nature and type of respiration.
7. Opioid overdose can suppress respiratory centres.
8. Increased intracranial pressure can leads to abnormal breathing
9. Neuromuscular diseses and polio can effect respiration by effecting the respiratory muscles.
10. CNS helps in respiration changes due to chemical changes in blood po2, pco2, ph etc.

CNS and immune system interlink

1. According to Pschychoimmunoneurology, autonomic nervous system i.e both sympathetic and parasympathetic nervous system, can play important role in controlling immune function of the body.
2. Blood brain barrier limits immune access to brain in normal physiological condition.
3. Microglia act as CNS macrophage and help in fighting against foreign particle in brain.
4. Many brain disorders occur due to autoimmune disorders of brain.

CNS and skeletal system interlink

1. Sympathetic and parasympsathic division of autonomic nervous system plays important role in bone metabolism by acting on osteoblasts or osteocytes or both.
2. Thus, CNS directly influences bone formation by acting on the bone cells.
3. Certain neuropeptides produced by CNS like CGRP, Substance P, VIP etc can influence bone cells.
4. Many hormones of hypothalamic-pituitary-bone axis play important role in bone mineral metabolism.
5. Research also shows that bone can send signals back to CNS via osteocalcin.
6. Mechanical stress on bone during exercise, can send signals to

brain via afferent nerves.

7. Newly, area of research is brain-bone axis in various bone diseases.

Interlinking of GIT with CVS

1. GIT and CVS are functionally and physiologically interconnected.

2. GIT depends upon CVS for blood supply, supply of nutrients, supply of oxygen etc.

3. GIT depends on CVS for blood flow.

4. GIT effects CVS through nutrients absorption.

5. Gut microbiota metabolizes food into compounds that can effect the hear and blood vessels.

6. GIT releases many hormones that effect CVS like GIP. GLP-1, ghrelin etc.

7. Several CVS illnesses can affect GIT, example heart failure leads to gut wall oedema etc.

8. GIT absorbs water, electrolytes, ions, glucose, amino acids and fatty acids into the ECF or blood and thus finally all these effect CVS activities directly and indirectly.

9. CVS supply blood to GIT organs and promotes their survival and help in the performing their normal function.

10. GIT help in absorption of nutrients like amino acid, glucose, [Na], [K], positive ions, negative ions, fatty acids, along H20, and thus help in maintenance of blood volume, and blood pressure and cardiac output.

11. GIT also absorbs [Na], [K], positive ions, negative ions, fatty acids, along with H20 and thus helps in maintenance of extracellular electrolyte balance, and thus electrolytes help in the cardiac electrical activities.

12. Liver produces albumin and plasma proteins which help in the maintenance of blood viscosity and this blood viscosity, maintains peripheral resistance and Blood pressure.

GIT and CNS interlinking

1. Autonomic nervous system has immense impact on GIT motility and secretion. Sympathetic stimulation and activity lowers GI secretion and Gi motility.

2. Parasympathetic activity and stimulation increase GI secretions and Gi motility.

3. Hypothalamus have two important centres i.e feeding centres (ventromedial nucleus) and satiety centre (lateral hypothalamus). These two centres together play important role in food intake or feeding behaviour, which is an important mechanism of gastrointestinal system.

4. CNS via autonomic nervous system controls GI hormones secretion like gastrin and cholecystokinin which control digestion and absorption.

5. Gut brain axis can influence appetite, satiety and food preference and also food intake.

6. Any dysregulation of gut brain axis contributes to various GIT disorders like irritable bowel syndrome, IBD, GERD etc.

7. Gut microbiota influences production of NTs, hormones etc that impact CNS function.

GIT and its interlinks with other systems

1. GIT secretes many GI hormones like Gastrin, CCK-PZ, VIP, secretin etc. which plays important role in Gi secretions and motility.

2. Respiratory system supplies fresh oxygen to GIT organs via blood and thus and there exists a lung-gut connections via neural and chemical signalling pathway.

3. Kidney excretes toxic substances like water, electrolytes, and metabolites of substrates which are absorbed via GIT system.

4. Blood supply nutrients, oxygen and necessary substates to GIT organs and GIT absorbs water, electrolytes, minerals and all other substances that form important composition of blood.

5. Immune system protects GI system from being attacked by foreign pathogen and GIT absorbs necessary substances, vitamins, minerals for immune system production.

6. GI system absorbs all necessary components, vitamins, minerals etc that are necessary for reproductive organs development, hormone generation, and overall activity of reproductive organs.

7. GI system helps in the absorption of calcium, phosphorus, amino acids, vitamins etc which play important role in bone formation and metabolism.

8. GI smooth muscle forms the muscular architecture of Gi system, Gi smooth muscle undergo contraction and relaxation and generate Gi movement under the guidance of Pace making system of intestine i.e interstitial cells of Cajal, which ultimately leads to peristalsis and other movement of git tract.

9. Special sense like visual impulse helps human beings to observe the quality of food intake, its smell, to differentiate it from toxins and thus help in the food intake.

Respiration and it interlink with other system

1. Respiration is under direct control of brain and autonomic nervous system.

2. CVS supply blood to respiratory system for gaseous exchange at lung.

3. Respiratory system supplies oxygenated blood to Gi system.

4. Respiratory system also helps in maintain blood pH, po2, pco2, etc which is necessary for all cells of the body including excretory system. Kidney senses PO2 and can produce erythropoietin to increase RBC production.

5. Respiratory system maintains blood PH, PO2, PCO2 etc and thus help in the physiological internal environment for all cells to work.

6. Respiratory system has airways smooth muscle, which contracts and relax and control the passage of air through it.

Excretory system and its interlinking with other system

1. Kidney plays important role in Blood pressure regulation, electrolyte balance, ph maintenance, RBC production etc.
2. Micturition reflex is under direct control from brain centres and renal blood flow is under control from autonomic nervous system.
3. Kidney filters blood, remove toxic products from blood, maintains blood volume and plasma osmolarity. Kidney also helps in RBC production by forming erythropoietin.
4. Immune system protects excretory organs from being attacked by foreign pathogen.
5. Kidney activates Vitamin D which along with PTH, and other hormones helps in calcium metabolism, and bone formation and metabolism.
6. Urinary tract consists of smooth muscle which contracts and relax to help in the passage of urine in urinary tract.
7. Many hormones like aldosterone, ADH, PTH, Vit D, ANP etc acts on the kidney and kidney also produce several hormones like renin, erythropoietin which play important role in blood pressure regulation and RBC production.

Thus, it can be stated that all systems of human physiological system depend on each other and thus they are interconnected directly or indirectly. Many systems get integrated together in performing a physiological task in human physiological system. They also play important role in internal homeostasis of the human body. Besides, due to any illness or in adverse situation if any system is affected, then other systems also try their best to help the human system to cop up with the new situation like in pregnancy, hypoxia, exercise, emergency, accidents, adverse life situations, etc. Also, in case of any illness or diseases, if one system is affected, it may affect other systems functions also as they are all interlinked, and hence there may multi systemic sign symptoms of a mono-systemic diseases or illness.

Mathematical modelling of unified theory of physiology

From the cardiac output equation in physiology,

It can be expressed as

Blood pressure= cardiac output. Peripheral resistance

Or, BP= CO. PR-----------------1 [where BP= mean arterial blood pressure,

CO=cardiac output,

PR= peripheral resistance]

From respiratory physiology,

R=Ventilation/perfusion ratio

=VA/Q $= \frac{VA}{Q}$ ---------------------------------------2

[where, VA = ventilation, Q= Perfusion, Ra= the ratio of ventilation and perfusion]

Or, Ra= $\frac{N.(VT-VD)}{Q} = \frac{N.(VT-VD)}{CO}$

[N = respiratory rate, VT= Tidal volume, VD= dead space volume, Q= perfusion=cardiac output=CO]

Also, from Bohr's equation of respiratory physiology,

$\frac{VD}{VT} = \frac{PaCO2-PECO2}{PaCO2}$ -------------3

[Where, VD= dead space volume,

VT= tidal volume, PaCo2= partial pressure of CO2 in arterial blood,

PECO2= partial pressure of CO2 in expired air]

Or, $\frac{VD}{VT} = 1 - \frac{PECO2}{Paco2}$

Or, $\frac{PECO2}{Paco2} = 1 - \frac{VD}{VT}$

Or, $\frac{PECO2}{Paco2} = \frac{VT-VD}{VT}$

Or, VT-VD $= \frac{PECO2.\ VT}{Paco2}$ -------------4

Now, comparing equation 2 and 4, we get,

Ra= $\frac{N.(VT-VD)}{Q} = \frac{N.PECO2.VT}{CO.PaCO2}$

Or, $CO = \frac{N.PECO2.VT}{Ra.Paco2}$ ------------------------5

Also,

From the mathematical physiology book by James Keener and James Sneyd, respiratory system equation 17.45, we get

VA/Q =Ra= $(RT.\ \{Wa - W0 + 4Z0[f(Wa) - f(W0)]\})/(Pio2 - Pao2)$ ----------------------6

[where, Pio2= partial pressure of the oxygen in inspired air,

PaO2= partial pressure of oxygen in alveolar air, f(W) = haemoglobin saturation function, Z0= total haemoglobin concentration, Wa = oxygen concentration in alveolar air, W0= oxygen concentration in blood input towards gaseous zone]

Now, comparing equation 5 and 6, we get

$CO = \frac{N.PECO2.VT}{Ra.Paco2} = \frac{N.PECO2.VT.(Pio2-Pao2)}{Paco2.\ RT.\ \{Wa-W0+4Z0[f(Wa)-f(W0)]\}}$ ----------------7

Now, comparing equation 1 and 7, we get,

BP= CO. PR

Or, BP $= \frac{N.PECO2.VT.(Pio2-Pao2)}{Paco2.\ RT.\ \{Wa-W0+4Z0[f(Wa)-f(W0)]\}}.PR$ ----------------8.

Also, from the cardiovascular physiology concept,

PR= Peripheral resistance= $8\eta l/\pi r4$ --------------------9 [η= viscosity of blood, l = length of the blood vessel, r=radius of the blood vessel]

Also, Re=Reynolds number= $\varrho vD/\eta$

[where, ϱ=density of blood, v= velocity of blood, D= diameter of blood vessel, η= viscosity of blood]

Or, $\eta = \varrho vD/Re$ ------------10

Now, comparing equation 9 and 10, we get,

PR=$8\eta l/\pi r4 = (16.L.\varrho.V)/(\pi r3.Re)$ ------------------11

Now, from Bernoulli's theorem in cardiovascular physiology, we get

$P + \frac{1}{2}.\varrho.v^2 + \varrho gh$ = constant= C

[Where, P= static pressure=BP=blood pressure, v=velocity of blood, g= acceleration due to gravity, h= height of the blood vessel, ϱ= density of blood flowing through blood vessel]

Or, $\frac{1}{2}.\varrho.v^2 = [C- P- \varrho gh]$

Or, $v=\sqrt{2(C-P-}\varrho gh)/\varrho$ ------------------12

Now, comparing equation 11 and 12, we get

$PR=\frac{8\eta l}{\pi r4} = \frac{16.L.\varrho.V}{\pi r3.Re} = \frac{16.L.\varrho.}{\pi r3.Re}\sqrt{2(C-P-}\varrho gh)/\varrho$

Or, $PR=\frac{16.L.\sqrt{2\varrho(C-P-}\varrho gh)}{\pi r3.Re}$ -------------------------13

Now, com;paring equation 8 and 13, we get,

$BP = \frac{N.PECO2.VT.(Pio2-Pao2)\frac{16.L.\sqrt{2\varrho(C-P-}\varrho gh)}{}}{Paco2.\ RT.\ \{Wa-W0+4Z0[f(Wa)-f(W0)]\}\pi r3.Re}$

$BP = \frac{N.PECO2.VT.(Pio2-Pao2)16.L.\sqrt{2\varrho(C-P-\varrho gh}}{Paco2.\ RT.\ \{Wa-W0+4Z0[f(Wa)-f(W0)]\}\pi r3.Re}$ --------------14

Now, from the concept of starling forces of renal physiology, we get

$GFR= Kf. [(P_{GC}-P_B)-(\pi_{GC}-\pi_B)]$ ------------15

[where, GFR= glomerular filtration rate, PGC= capillary hydrostatic pressure, PB= hydrostatic pressure in Bowman's capsule, π_{GC} =glomerular capillary oncotic pressure, π_B= oncotic pressure of Bowmans capsule]

Also, PGC= K1. BP, [where. K1= constant and BP= systemic arterial pressure]

Or, $GFR= Kf. [(K1.\ BP-P_B)-(\pi_{GC}-\pi_B)]$

Or, $\frac{GFR}{Kf} = K1.BP-P_B-\pi_{GC}+\pi_B$

or, $K1.BP-P_B-\pi_{GC}+\pi_B = \frac{GFR}{Kf}$

or, $K1.\ BP=\frac{GFR}{Kf} +P_B+ \pi_{GC} - \pi_B$

OR, $BP = 1/k1\{\frac{GFR}{Kf} +P_B+ \pi_{GC} - \pi_B\}$

or, $BP = \frac{\frac{GFR}{Kf} +PB+ \pi GC - \pi B}{K1}$ -------------------------16

Comparing equations 14 and 16, we get,

$$\frac{\frac{GFR}{Kf} + \text{PB} + \pi\text{GC} - \pi\text{B}}{K1} = \frac{N.PECO2.VT.(Pio2 - Pao2)16.L.\sqrt{2\varrho(C - BP - \varrho gh}}{Paco2.\ RT.\ \{Wa - W0 + 4Z0[f(Wa) - f(W0)]\}\pi r3.Re}$$

Or, $\frac{\frac{GFR}{Kf} + \text{PB} + \pi\text{GC} - \pi\text{B}}{K1} = \frac{N.PECO2.VT.(Pio2 - Pao2)16.L.\sqrt{2\varrho(C - BP - \varrho gh)}}{Paco2.\ RT.\ \{Wa - W0 + 4Z0[f(Wa) - f(W0)]\}\pi r3.Re}$ --17

Now, from the concept of hematology,

ϱ= density of blood = (1-H). ϱp+ H. ϱ_{RBC} ------------------18

[Where, H= hematocrit value, ϱRBC= density of RBC cells, ϱp= density of plasma]

Also, density of plasma = ϱp is given by an equation which is used for clinical studies,

[TP]=a(ϱp-b)

Or, $\frac{[TP]}{a}$ = ϱp-b

Or, ϱp = b+$\frac{[TP]}{a}$ -------------19

[where, [TP]= Plasma protein concertation, ϱp = density of plasma, a, b = constants]

Now, comparing equation 19 and 18 and 17, we get,

$$\frac{\frac{GFR}{Kf} + \text{PB} + \pi\text{GC} - \pi\text{B}}{K1} = \frac{N.PECO2.VT.(Pio2 - Pao2)16.L.\sqrt{2[(\text{b}+\frac{[TP]}{a})(1-\text{H}).+ \text{H}.\varrho\text{RB}](C - BP - \varrho gh)}}{Paco2.\ RT.\ \{Wa - W0 + 4Z0[f(Wa) - f(W0)]\}\pi r3.Re}$$ ---------20

Now, we know,

[TP] = $\frac{\text{total plasma protein}}{\text{plasma volume}} = \frac{TPP}{PV}$ ------21 or, PV= TPP/[TP]

Now, from the equation of plasma osmolarity, we get

Calculated Plasma osmolarity = P_{Oc}= 2. [Na+] + [glucose]/18 + [BUN]/6 --------------22

[Where, [Na+] = plasma sodium ion concentration,

[Glucose]= plasma concentration of glucose

[BUN] = plasma blood urea nitrogen]

activity, α1 = constant related to sympathetic activity, β1 = constant related to parasympathic activity, Sa = sympathetic activity, Psa= parasympathetic activity]

Now, comparing equation 32 and 31, we get

$$\frac{\frac{GFR}{Kf}+\text{PB}+\pi\text{GC}-\pi\text{B}}{K1} = (N.PECO2.VT.(Pio2 - Pao2)16.L.\sqrt{}(2[(\text{b}+[(\text{f1}(\text{PI},\text{LF},\text{KF}).\ (\text{POM}-\text{OG}-\ -\text{f2}(\text{Hc},\text{Hi},\text{Fg})/18-[\text{f3}(\text{LF},\text{KF},\text{Pm})]/6))/(2.\text{f4}\ (\text{FNa},\text{KF},\text{Ald},\text{ANP})\ )]/a)(1-\text{H}).+\text{H}.\varrho\text{RB}](C-BP-)\ \varrho\text{gh}))/(Re.Paco2.\ RT.\ \{Wa-W0+4Z0[f(Wa)-f(W0)]\}\pi Sa.Sa.Sa\ (\text{ro}/\text{Sa}-\alpha1\ +\ \beta1.\text{Psa}/\text{Sa})3\ )$$

---------------------------------equation 33

Now, let's discuss about bone physiology. The measure of bone health is given by bone mineral density (BMD) as estimated by DEXA scan. Now, according to latest literature, Bone health depends upon various factors like gene, age, hormones, nutrition, and lifestyle. That means good nutrition diet rich in calcium, protein, and phosphorus and vitamins like Vitamin D can play important role in bone formation. At the same time, various hormones responsible for bone metabolism like Vitamin D, PTH, cortisol, thyroid hormone, calcitonin, etc can play important role in osteoblastic and osteoclastic resorption, that effect the bone mineral density.

Besides, genetic makeup i.e gene and age of the subject also plays important role in bone health maintenance. Now, literature shows that sympathetic and parasympathetic nervous system also can affect bone health. Sympathetic activity and stimulation lead to increase in osteoclastic activity and bone resorption and decrease bone formation whereas parasympathetic activity effect the bone heath by increasing in osteoblastic activity.

Hence, we can express bone health or bone mineral density (BMD) = f5(gene, age, HCa2+, Dn) + f6(Psa) – f7(Sa)

[where, Dn= diet and nutrition rich in calcium, protein etc,

Hca2= all hormones for calcium metabolism,

Psa= parasympathetic activity,

Sa = sympathetic activity]

Or, f7(Sa) = f5(gene, age, HCa2+, Dn) + f6(Psa) – BMD

Or, Sa= f_7^{-1} [f5(gene, age, HCa2+, Dn) + f6(Psa)–**BMD**] =F1(**BMD**) (suppose)----------------------34

Let's focus on reproductive activity of human physiological system. Both sympathetic activity and parasympathetic activity can affect the reproductive activity in different way. Hence, RA = reproductive activity can be expressed as sum of the function of

F8(Hr, Dn, Age, gene, life style, overall health) + f9(Sa) + F10(Psa)

Or, RA= f8(Hr, Dn, Age, gene, life style, overall health) -f9(Sa) + f10(Psa)

[where, RA = reproductive activity,

Hr= reproductive hormones,

Dn= diet and nutrition,

Sa= sympathetic activity,

Psa= parasympathetic activity]

Or, f9(Sa) = {f8(Hr, Dn, Age, gene, life style, overall health) + f10(Psa)-RA}

Or, Sa= f_9^{-1}{f8(Hr, Dn, Age, gene, life style, overall health) + f10(Psa)-**RA**}

= F2(**RA**) (suppose)--------------35

Now, lets focus on the effect of sympathetic and parasympathetic activity on Gastrointestinal tract motility and secretion (GIms). Sympathetic stimulation and activity decreases GI motility and secretion and this its action is inhibitory to GIT. On the other hand, parasympathetic is stimulatory to GI motility and secretion.

Hence, [GI m,s] = f11(GIh, Lof,, Ir) -f12(Sa)+ f13(Psa) [where, GIh=gi hormones, lof=local factors, Ir= intrinsic regulatory factors]

Or, f12(Sa) = f11(GIh, Lof,, Ir) + f13(Psa) - [GI m,s]

Or, Sa= f_{12}^{-1} {f11 (GIh, Lof, Ir) + f13 (Psa) - [**GI m,s**] }

Or, Sa= F3([**GI m,s**])(suppose)---------------36

Now let us consider effect of sympathetic and parasympathetic activity on the immune system of the body.

IA = f14(Psa)-f15(Sa) + f16{gene, age, Dn, Ls}

Or, f15(Sa) = f14(Psa) + f16(gene, age, Dn, Ls)-IA

Or, Sa = f_{15}^{-1} {f14(Psa) + f16(gene, age, Dn, Ls)-**IA**}

Or, Sa= F4(**IA**) (suppose)---------------37

Or, IA + f15(Sa) -f16{gene, age, Dn, Ls} = f14(Psa)

Or, Psa = f_{14}^{-1} {IA + f15(Sa) -f16(gene, age, Dn, Ls)} = F5(**IA**) (suppose)

[Where, Dn= diet and nutrition, Ls=lifestyle changes, IA = immune activity]

If we look into the effect of sympathetic and parasympathetic stimulatory activity on cognitive function, it can be expressed that,

C_f= cognitive function = f17(Gene, Ls, Bh, Age, Edu, NB) + f18(PSa)-f(Sa) = Cf

Or, f19(Sa) = f17(Gene, Ls, Bh, Age, Edu, NB) + f18(PSa) -Cf

Or, Sa = f_{19}^{-1} {f17(Gene, Ls, Bh, Age, Edu, NB) + f18(PSa) -**Cf**}

Or, Sa= F5 (**Cf**)

Also, f18(PSa)= Cf -f17(Gene, Ls, Bh, Age, Edu, NB)+ f19(Sa)

Or Psa = F6(**Cf**) (suppose)-----------------------38

[where, Ls= lifestyle changes, Bh= brain health, NB= neurotransmitter in brain]

Now, considering equation 33, 34, 45, 36, 37, 38, we get,

$$\frac{\frac{GFR}{Kf} + \text{PB} + \pi\text{GC} - \pi\text{B}}{K1} = (N.PECO2.VT.(Pio2 - Pao2)16.L.\sqrt{(}2[(\text{b} +$$

$[(\mathbf{f1(PI, LF, KF)}.\ (\mathbf{POM - OG - \ -f2(Hc, Hi, Fg)/18 -}$
$\mathbf{[f3(LF, KF, Pm)]/6))/(2.f4\ (FNa, KF, Ald, ANP)}\ )]/a)(1 -$
$\mathrm{H}). + \mathrm{H}.\varrho\mathrm{RB}](C - \boldsymbol{BP}-)\ \varrho\mathrm{gh}))/(Re.Paco2.\ RT.\ \{Wa - W0 +$
$4Z0[f(Wa) -$
$f(W0)]\}\pi.\mathrm{F1}(\mathbf{BMD}).\mathrm{F2}(\mathbf{RA}).\mathrm{F3}(\ [\mathbf{GI\ m, s}]\ )\mathrm{Psa}.\mathrm{F6}(\mathbf{Cf})\mathrm{F5}(\ \mathbf{IA}).\ (\mathrm{ro}/$
$(\mathrm{Sa.Psa}) - \alpha 1/\mathrm{Psa}\ \ + \ \beta 1.1/\mathrm{Sa})3\ \ )$

------------------39

Now, lets suppose $\{Wa - W0 + 4Z0[f(Wa) - f(W0)]\}$ = **F7(Hbs, [O2])** (suppose)---- 40

That means, it is a function of Hb saturation and oxygen concentration. Hence, Equation 39 and 40, becomes

$$\frac{\frac{GFR}{Kf} + \mathrm{PB} + \pi\mathrm{GC} - \pi\mathrm{B}}{K1} = (N.PECO2.VT.(Pio2 - Pao2)16.L.\sqrt{}(2[(\mathrm{b} +$$
$$[(\mathbf{f1(PI, LF, KF)}.\ (\mathbf{POM - OG - \ -f2(Hc, Hi, Fg)/18 -}$$
$$\mathbf{[f3(LF, KF, Pm)]/6))/(2.f4\ (FNa, KF, Ald, ANP)}\ )]/a)(1 -$$
$$\mathrm{H}). + \mathrm{H}.\varrho\mathrm{RB}](C - \boldsymbol{BP}-)\ \varrho\mathrm{gh}))/$$
$$(Re.Paco2.\{\ \mathbf{F7(\ Hbs, [O2])}\}.RT.\ \pi.\mathrm{F1}(\mathbf{BMD}).\mathrm{F2}(\mathbf{RA}).\mathrm{F3}$$
$$(\ [\mathbf{GI\ m, s}]\ )\mathrm{Psa}.\mathrm{F6}(\mathbf{Cf})\mathrm{F5}(\ \mathbf{IA}).\ (\mathrm{ro}/(\mathrm{Sa.Psa}) - \alpha 1/\mathrm{Psa}$$
$$+ \ \beta 1.1/\mathrm{Sa})3\ \ )$$

----------------------------------41

Now, according to Weir equations,

BMR=Basal metabolic rate= (3.941. VO2+ 1.106. VCO2). 1440 ------------------42

[where, VO2= oxygen consumption in liters /min

VCO2= CO2 consumption]

Also, RQ= Respiratory quotient= VCO2/ VO2-----43

Also, from alveolar gas equation, we get

PAO2=FiO2(Patm-PH20)-PaCo2/RQ ----------------44

Also, from Fickes principle of cardiac output measurement,

CO=$\frac{VO2}{CaO2-CvO2}$ --------------------45

Now, comparing equations, 42, 43, 44, 45, we get,

$$PaCO2=\frac{\frac{BMR}{1440}-3.941.VO2)\{Fio2(Patm-PH20)-PAo2\}}{1.106.\boldsymbol{CO}.\{CaO2-Cvo2\}} \text{ -----------------------46}$$

Now, comparing, equation 46 and 41, we get,

$$\frac{\frac{GFR}{Kf}+PB+(ngc-nb)\mathbf{RT}}{K1}=$$

$$N.PECO2.VT.(Pi-Pa)16.1.106.\boldsymbol{CO}.\{\boldsymbol{CaO2}-\boldsymbol{Cvo2}\}\,L.$$

$$\sqrt{2[(b+\frac{\left[\frac{f1(PI,LF,KF).(POM-OG--\frac{f2(Hc,Hi,Fg)}{18}-\frac{[f3(LF,KF,Pm)]}{6})}{2.f4(FNa,KF,Ald,ANP)}\right]}{a})(1-H).+H.\varrho RB](C-\boldsymbol{BP}-\varrho gh)}\Big/$$

$$Re\frac{BMR}{1440}-3.941.VO2)\{Fio2(Patm-PH20)-PAo2\}..\{\mathbf{F7}(\mathbf{Hbs},[\mathbf{O2}]i\}.RT.\,\pi.F1(\mathbf{BMD}).F2(\mathbf{RA}).$$

$$F3([\mathbf{GI\ m,s}]).Psa.F6(\mathbf{Cf}).F5(\mathbf{IA}).\left(\frac{ro}{Sa.Psa}-\frac{\alpha 1}{Psa}+\beta 1.\frac{1}{Sa}\right)3$$

-----------------------47

Now,

1.Here, GFR, KF= a parameter of excretory system,

2. CO, BP, ro, L, Re = they are important parameters of cardiovascular system,

3. VT, reflects respiratory system parameter.

4.N=respiratory rate can be expressed as (RR0+ α2. Sa-β2. Psa)

= **[f (BSa, PO2, PCO2, PH, T) + α2. Sa-β2. Psa**]

=depends on various biophysical parameters, brainstem activity, sympathetic and parasympathetic activity.

5. H= hematocrit value= a parameter of haemato physiology.

ϱ= blood density = a parameter of blood physziolgy

6. IA = Immune system activity

7. BMD= Bone health activity

8. RA= Reproductive system activity,

9. GIm,s = Gastro intestinal physiology and git motility and secretion

10. Cf = cognitive function of brain

11. BMR = parameter of metabolism

12. In this part of equation,

$$\frac{\mathbf{f1(PI,LF,KF).\ (POM-OG-}-\frac{\mathbf{f2(Hc,Hi,Fg)}}{\mathbf{18}}-\frac{\mathbf{[f3(LF,KF,Pm)]}}{\mathbf{6}}\mathbf{)}}{\mathbf{2.f4\ (FNa,KF,Ald,ANP)}},$$

here Hc, Hi, etc reflect all catabolic hormones, insulin, beside other hormones are also included in this function and these are part of endocrine system.

13. Sa, Psa etc reflects autonomic nervous system parameters.

14. Beside other parameters like genetics, feeding behavior, hemoglobin saturation curve all are involved in this equation.

15. RT reflect product of gas constant and temperature in absolute scale.

$$1/RT = \frac{2.303}{Em.F}\log.\ \frac{Pk.Ko+Pna.NaOut+Pcl.Cli+\cdots.}{k.Ki+Pna.Nai+Pcl.Clo+\cdots..} \text{ ------------------------48}$$

[Where, Pk= permeability of potassium, Kao= potassium concentration outside etc

Em=RMP, F = faraday constant]

Hence, it can be seen that this equation unifies all systems of human physiology starting from biophysical parameters, RMP, CVS, CNS, Brain, Immune system, blood physiology, bone physiology, reproductive system, excretory system, GIT, excretory system, etc and this is the mathematical model of unified theory of physiology. This equation integrates all important parameters of all physiological systems of the human body and hence, it is the ultimate theory of grand unification of physiology. Some of the complex relationships of physiological parameters are expressed in the form of function of several parameters as many of functional correlation has not been discovered or are very complex to define in a single equation.

Now as per reference number 4, and in my paper "**Unification of Electromagnetism, Gravity and Quantum Mechanics in Human**

Physiological System" I have already shown that how various parameters like electromagnetism, gravity and quantum mechanics can be correlated under the platform of cardiovascular system, neurophysiology. From the equation of my paper, it can be expressed as

$K_1.\ K_2[\ 1 + \{\ \sqrt{\mu}\ a^3/\ (4\mathbf{B}\ r_1R1.\ K_3^2.\ D^{2N3}).\ d^2V/dt^2\ \ -1\}^{\ 1/N4}]^{\ N1+N2} + Re.r2.\sqrt{\boldsymbol{h}\pi}\frac{}{32\sqrt{\lambda\varrho}}\ + \mathbf{G}.M_E.H.R_e.\pi r^4.\ \sqrt{\pi\lambda\varrho}\ /16.(R_E{+}H)^2\sqrt{h}\ \ - C.R_e.\pi r^4 \sqrt{\pi\lambda}/\ 16.\sqrt{\varrho h}\ \ {=}0$

Or, $Re.r2.\sqrt{\boldsymbol{h}\pi}\frac{}{32\sqrt{\lambda\varrho}}\ =\ C.R_e.\pi r^4\ \sqrt{\pi\lambda}/\ 16.\sqrt{\varrho h}\ -\ K_1.\ K_2[\ 1 + \{\ \sqrt{\mu}\ a^3/\ (4\mathbf{B}\ r_1R1.\ K_3^2.\ D^{2N3}).\ d^2V/dt^2\ \ -1\}^{\ 1/N4}]^{\ N1+N2}\ \ -\ \mathbf{G}.M_E.H.R_e.\pi r^4.\ \sqrt{\pi\lambda\varrho}\ /16.(R_E{+}H)^2\sqrt{h}$ -----------------48

Or, $Re=\frac{32\sqrt{\lambda\varrho}}{r2.\sqrt{\boldsymbol{h}\pi}}[\ C.R_e.\pi r^4\ \sqrt{\pi\lambda}/\ 16.\sqrt{\varrho h}\ -\ K_1.\ K_2[\ 1 + \{\ \sqrt{\mu}\ a^3/\ (4\mathbf{B}\ r_1R1.\ K_3^2.\ D^{2N3}){-}\ \ \mathbf{G}.M_E.H.R_e.\pi r^4.\ \ \sqrt{\pi\lambda\varrho}\ \ /16.(R_E{-}H)^2\sqrt{h}\ \ ]$ 49

[Where, Re = Reynolds number
B= strength of magnetic field of the neuron,
h=Planck constant,
G= Gravitational constant
λ=De-Broglie's wavelength of blood
$\varrho = density\ of\ the\ blood$
d^2V/dt^2 = rate of change of voltage of neuronal membrane]

Now, in equation 47 also, there is a Reynolds number, we can substitute Reynolds number with the equation 49, and then we can create a new equation of **unified theory of physiology**, along with unification of **gravity, electromagnetism and quantum mechanics**. This is because the new equation has **B**, which is the strength of magnetic field, **G**, which gravitational constant, and **h,** which is Planck constant, which is an important parameter of quantum mechanics. Since, this equation also unifies gravity and electromagnetism along with parameters of all physiological systems, it can also be termed as **Grand Unified theory of Physiology**.

Hence, the final equation becomes the **Grand unified theory of physiology**, where along with physiological parameters of all systems, gravity, electromagnetism and quantum mechanics has also been integrated.

Physiological and clinical Importance of the unified theory

This theory shows that all physiological system can be correlated and they are interdependent in each other in maintaining of physiological stability and maintaining physiological state of the body. That means every physiological mechanism that occurs in human body in any system has some effect on other system directly or indirectly. Hence, all physiological systems of human body are interlinked or interdependent on each other and all of them can be correlated to one another so as to perform the normal physiological activities of the human body. It also means to say if one system is involved in doing some physiological activities in inside human body, the other systemic changes will also occur to some extent directly or indirectly. This also prove that if any pathology occurs in human body, the systems will be affected as well as they are all interlinked. This theory bridges all systemic parameters of all the systems including biophysical parameters starting from cellular mechanism, genetic level to the complex network of human brain and other systems. It can also predict the outcome of the change in other systems of the body if one of the systems is involved in any physiological activities. It also shows that if any pathological change occurs in any system or any system is affected by any diseases, other systems of the human body will be affected. Thus, in any diseases process, if one system is involved, other systems will be involved or other parameters of other systems will be affected and it also explains the multiple sign systems of a one systemic disease. That means if one systemic disease occurs in human body, multiple sign symptoms may appear that involve other systems of the body, beyond the original system of the diseases. That also proves that any latent diseases if occurs, others systemic parameters should be checked so that the diseases can be diagnosed at early stage. In case of a single systemic or organ diseases, other systemic parameters and functions can be affected, which may help in easy diagnosis of the illness or pathology. This change of parameters may be due to adjustment that occurs in the body in response to pathology or that may be due to the systemic interlink of all the biological systems of human body. Hence, it also proves that if the cause of ill ness is removed then all the parameters will come to normal side after total cure of the illness. Besides, this unified theory also proves that our human physiological system work by involving all systems together, if any one of the systems are involved, it can affect the other systems directly or indirectly. In the last part of the theory, I have unified gravity, electromagnetism and quantum mechanics along with the systemic unified theory and the final equation shows unification of all systems of physiology with the theories of physics. This theory may open up new horizon and further research can be done on the unified theory of physiology. The theory can be applied to explain outcome in diseases and illness. This theory can form a conceptual backbone for medical education and biological education. This theory can be pathfinder in systems biology research and can be important for science, medicine and system thinking. This theory can show us the path towards mathematical modelling of diseases and illness.

References

1. Text book of medical physiology by Arthur Guyton and JE Hall
2. Ganongs review of medical physiology.
3. Nature design of human physiological system
4. (Hematological system) by Dr. **Omkar Prasad Baidya** on 2025, published by Prachi digital publisher, Nainital.
5. **Omkar Prasad Baidya**. Unification of Electromagnetism, Gravity and Quantum Mechanics in Human Physiological System. Volume - 13 | Issue - 08 | August - 2024 |

References

1. Text book of medical physiology by Arthur Guyton and JE Hall
2. Ganongs review of medical physiology.
3. Nature design of human physiological system
4. (Hematological system) by Dr. **Omkar Prasad Baidya** on 2025, published by Prachi digital publisher, Nainital.
5. **Omkar Prasad Baidya**. Unification of Electromagnetism, Gravity and Quantum Mechanics in Human Physiological System. Volume - 13 | Issue - 08 | August - 2024 |

References

1. Text book of medical physiology by Arthur Guyton and JE Hall
2. Ganongs review of medical physiology.
3. Nature design of human physiological system
4. (Hematological system) by Dr. **Omkar Prasad Baidya** on 2025, published by Prachi digital publisher, Nainital.
5. **Omkar Prasad Baidya**. Unification of Electromagnetism, Gravity and Quantum Mechanics in Human Physiological System. Volume - 13 | Issue - 08 | August - 2024 |